PEST - FREE NATURALLY

HOME REMEDIES FOR EVERY BUG BATTLE

MISTI COYLE

ISBN:

978-1-966968-28-3 (eBook)
978-1-966968-29-0 (Paperback)

Published by:

OWL® PUBLISHERS

www.owlpublishers.com

360 S Market St, San Jose, CA 95113,

United States.

Printed in the United States of America

ABOUT THE BOOK

Pest-Free Naturally: Home Remedies for Every Bug Battle is your friendly, down-to-earth guide to getting rid of common household pests without harsh chemicals. With a warm, natural tone and decades of pest control know-how, Misti Coyle walks you through easy DIY solutions for ants, roaches, flies, fleas, bed bugs, and more—complete with bonus tips and prevention strategies to keep your home bug-free for good.

Table of Content

CHAPTER 1
ANTS — THE TINY MARCHING ARMY

Ants are everywhere — tiny, organized, and relentless. They march through your kitchen and invade your pantry like they own the place. But guess what? They don't. You do. Let's send those little invaders packing, naturally.

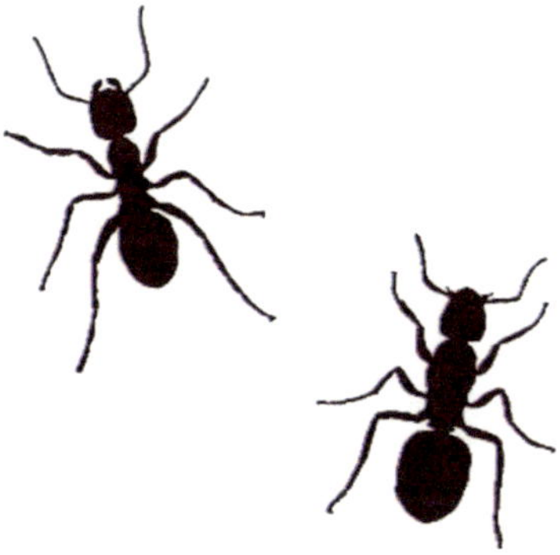

Why They Come:
Ants are attracted to food crumbs, sugary spills, and open access to water sources.

Natural Remedies:

- **Vinegar Spray:** Equal parts white vinegar and water destroys their scent trail.
- **Cinnamon:** Sprinkle ground cinnamon at entry points. Ants won't cross it.
- **Lemon Juice:** Breaks their trails and acts as a natural deterrent.
- **Boric Acid + Sugar Paste:** Mix to attract and eliminate the colony (keep away from pets and kids).

Lifestyle & Prevention Tips:

- Wipe counters and sweep floors daily.
- Seal food in airtight containers.
- Take out the trash regularly.
- Trim back outdoor plants touching your house.

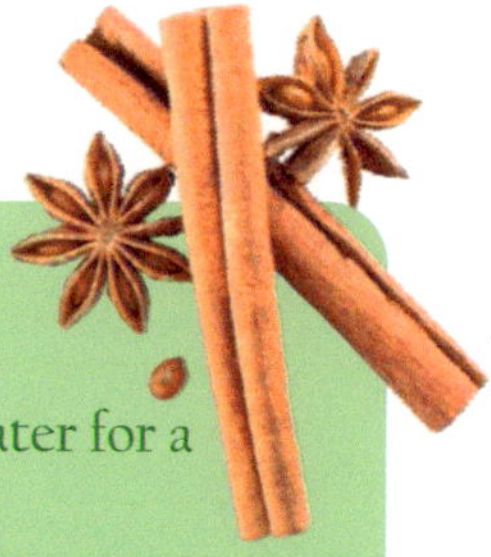

Bonus Tips:

- Use a mixture of peppermint essential oil and water for a pleasant-smelling ant repellent.
- Caulk around doors and windows to block entry.
- Ant-proof pet food bowls with a shallow dish of water underneath.

When to Call a Pro:

If ants are visible during the day, multiply fast, or you notice droppings and egg casings, it's time to call in professionals for a thorough treatment.

CHAPTER 2
ROACHES — THE RELENTLESS NIGHTCRAWLERS

Nothing causes a bigger shudder than turning on the lights and seeing roaches scatter. These resilient bugs thrive in hidden places and multiply quickly—but you've got natural power on your side.

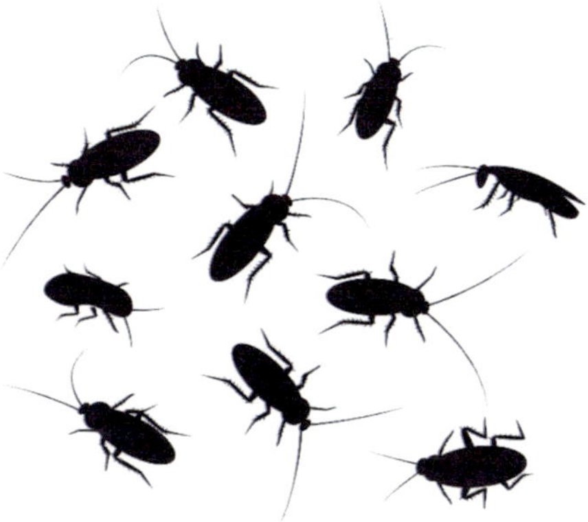

Why They Come:
Food, water, and shelter. Roaches love dark, damp areas like kitchens and bathrooms.

Natural Remedies:

- **Baking Soda + Sugar Trap:** Equal parts mixed and placed in shallow lids.
- **Bay Leaves:** Crushed and scattered in cabinets to repel roaches.
- **Diatomaceous Earth:** Safe for people and pets—sprinkle under sinks and behind appliances.
- **Essential Oils:** Eucalyptus and peppermint oil work wonders. Spray diluted versions around baseboards.

Lifestyle & Prevention Tips:

- Fix leaky pipes and dry out sinks at night.
- Don't leave dirty dishes out overnight.
- Empty trash daily.
- Deep clean behind the fridge and stove monthly.

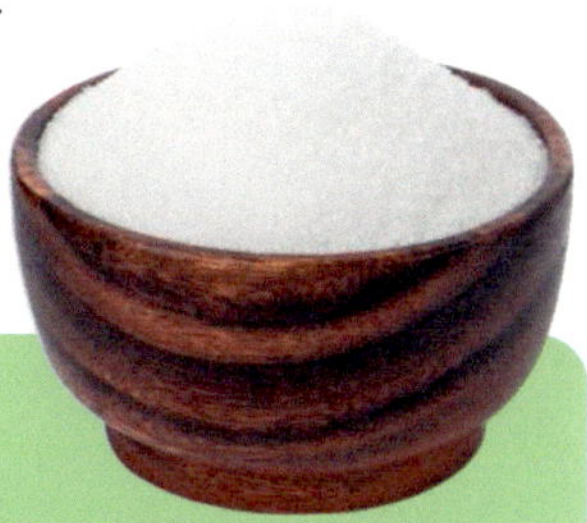

Bonus Tips:

- Declutter paper and cardboard—roaches love nesting in them.
- Place cucumber slices in hotspots; they hate the scent.
- Keep pantry staples in glass or hard plastic containers.

When to Call a Pro:

If roaches are visible during the day, multiply fast, or you notice droppings and egg casings, it's time to call in professionals for a thorough treatment

CHAPTER 3
FRUIT FLIES — THE TINY FLYERS OF DOOM

They're not dangerous, but they are so annoying. Fruit flies are sneaky and love your kitchen as much as you do. Time to end the fruit fly fiesta.

Why They Come:
Overripe fruit, food scraps, and drains are prime fruit fly real estate.

Natural Remedies:

- **Apple Cider Vinegar Trap:** Mix ACV with dish soap in a small bowl. Cover with plastic wrap and poke holes.
- **Red Wine Trap:** They can't resist it. Same setup as the ACV trap.
- **Basil Plant:** Natural repellent for counters and windowsills.
- **Boiling Water:** Flush kitchen drains regularly.

Lifestyle & Prevention Tips:

- Keep fruit in the fridge.
- Empty and clean trash cans frequently.
- Clean sink strainers and disposals with baking soda and vinegar.

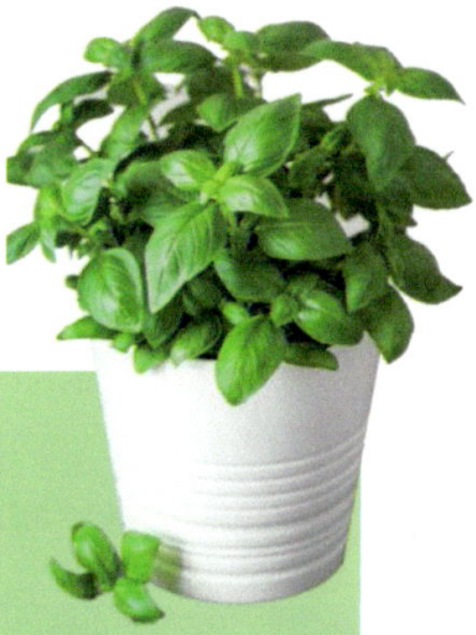

Bonus Tips:

- Wash fruit as soon as you bring it home.
- Use a fan to blow them away from prep areas.
- Dry out sponge holders and under-sink areas.

When to Call a Pro:

If fruit flies keep returning despite eliminating breeding grounds, a pro can inspect hidden sources and help you break the cycle.

CHAPTER 4
MOSQUITOES — THE BUZZING BLOODSUCKERS

They bite, they whine, and they ruin evenings. These pests are annoying at best and dangerous at worst—but don't worry, you're about to turn your home into a no-fly zone.

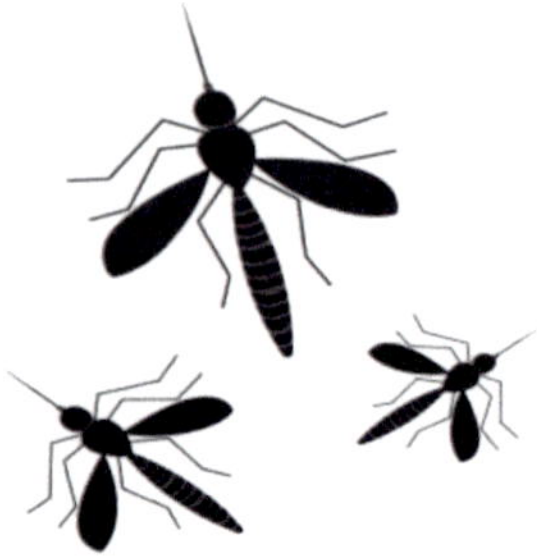

Why They Come:
Standing water and shady, humid areas are mosquito havens.

Natural Remedies:

- **Citronella Candles:** Great for patios and entryways.
- **Lavender Oil Spray:** Mix with water and spritz on skin and clothes.
- **Neem Oil:** Works as a body-safe deterrent in small amounts.
- **Coffee Grounds:** Sprinkle in standing water to prevent larvae growth.

Lifestyle & Prevention Tips:

- Empty birdbaths, planters, and pet bowls often.
- Use fans in outdoor areas—mosquitoes hate wind.
- Install screens on windows and doors.
- Mow tall grass and trim shrubs regularly.

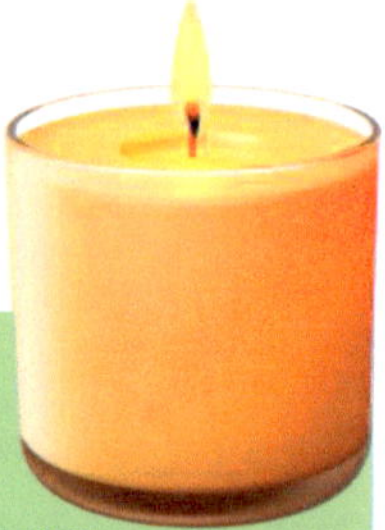

Bonus Tips:

- Plant mosquito-repelling herbs: basil, mint, rosemary.
- Use yellow bug lights outdoors.
- Hang mosquito netting over outdoor sitting areas.

When to Call a Pro:
If outdoor infestations persist or you live near wetlands, call professionals for fogging or parricide options.

CHAPTER 5
FLIES — THE UNWANTED HOUSEGUESTS

They land on your food, your face, your walls—and they've been everywhere else first. It's time to give flies the boot with fresh, chemical-free tactics.

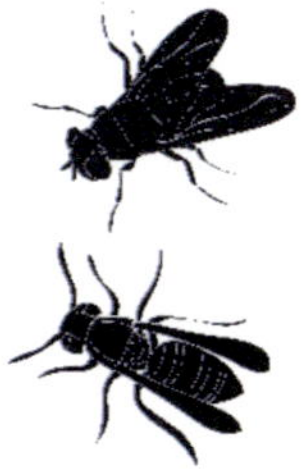

Why They Come:
Open trash, pet waste, food spills, and even houseplants can invite flies.

Natural Remedies:

- **Clove-Stuffed Lemon:** Cut a lemon and stud it with whole cloves—flies hate it.
- **DIY Fly Traps:** Apple cider vinegar + dish soap in a jar with plastic wrap and holes.
- **Cucumber Slices:** Place on counters and window sills.
- **Eucalyptus Oil:** Use in a diffuser or cotton balls placed in corners.

Lifestyle & Prevention Tips:

- Keep trash bins sealed and clean.
- Clean up crumbs and spills quickly.
- Pick up pet waste daily from the yard.

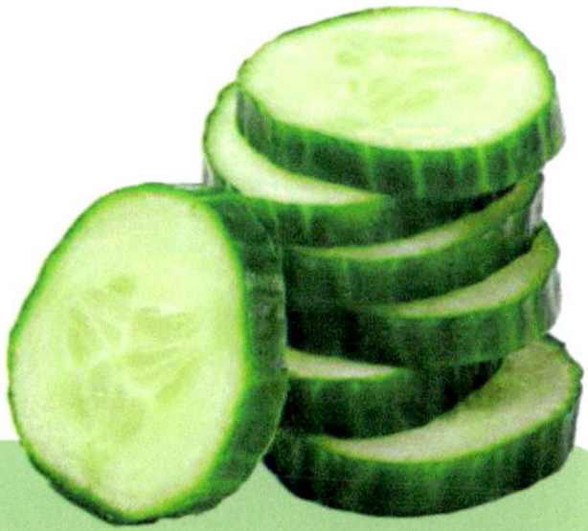

Bonus Tips:

- Hang clear plastic bags filled with water by doors and windows.
- Use fine mesh screens on all entry points.
- Clean drains with baking soda + vinegar.

When to Call a Pro:
If flies are persistent despite cleaning and trapping, there may be a hidden breeding source. Pros can inspect and eliminate it.

CHAPTER 6
FLEAS — THE HOPPING MENACE

They hop, they bite, and they turn pets into itchy messes. Fleas are tough—but not tougher than you.

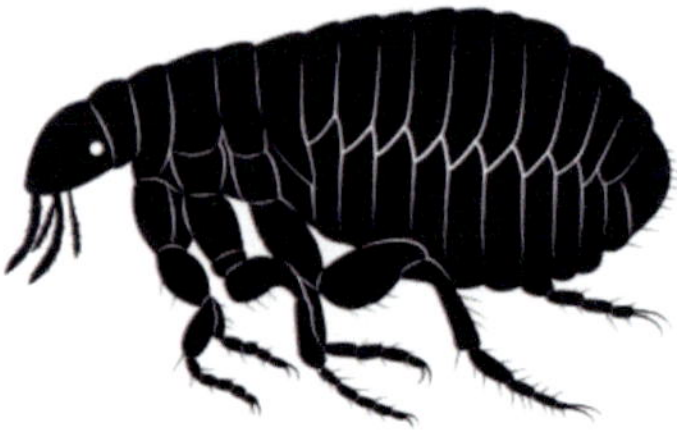

Why They Come:
They ride in on pets, clothing, or wildlife and settle into carpets and bedding.

Natural Remedies:

- **Salt or Baking Soda:** Sprinkle on carpets, let sit, and then vacuum.
- **Lemon Spray:** Slice lemon into hot water, steep overnight, and spray on pet bedding.
- **Cedar Chips:** Place under pet beds and furniture.
- **Apple Cider Vinegar Rinse:** Add to pet's bathwater (check with your vet first).

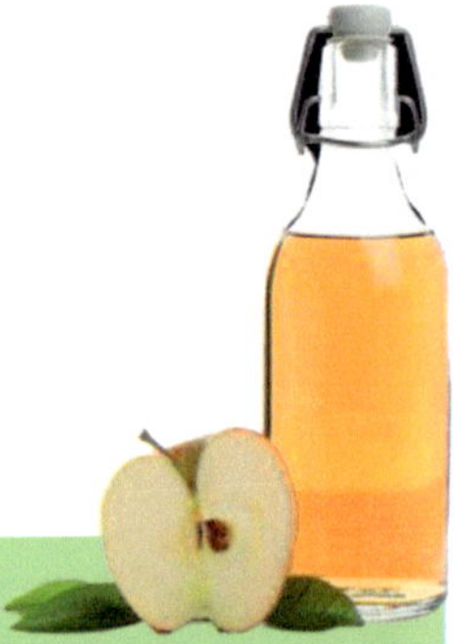

Lifestyle & Prevention Tips:

- Bathe and comb pets weekly.
- Wash bedding in hot water.
- Vacuum carpets and furniture often.

Bonus Tips:

- Use flea combs with a bowl of soapy water to drown them.
- Keep lawns trimmed and avoid tall grass.
- Place flea traps (light + dish soap) near pet resting areas.

When to Call a Pro:
If home treatments fail or infestation spreads quickly, professional flea treatment is essential.

CHAPTER 7
SPIDERS — THE CREEPY CRAWLERS

Spiders give most people the heebie-jeebies. While they help control other bugs, you probably don't want them hanging out in your shower or closet. Let's get them out—kindly and naturally.

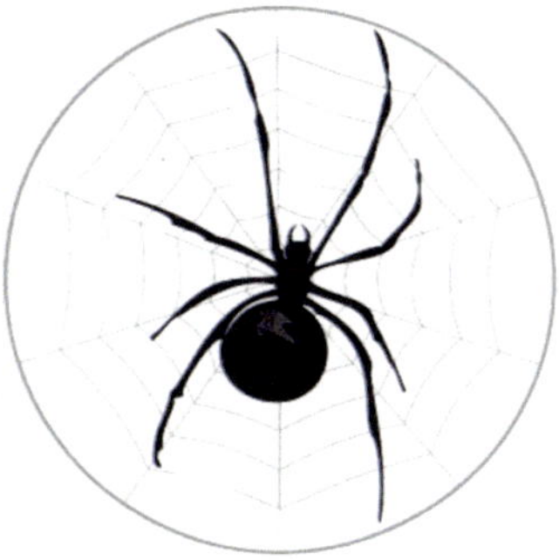

Why They Come:
Spiders follow other bugs—their food. So, a spider problem often means another bug problem too.

Natural Remedies:

- **White Vinegar Spray:** Mix with water and spray corners, baseboards, and under furniture.
- **Peppermint Oil:** A few drops in water makes a great spray repellent.
- **Citrus Peels:** Rub window sills and door frames with lemon or orange peels.
- **Diatomaceous Earth:** Spread lightly around entry points.

Lifestyle & Prevention Tips:

- Declutter! Spiders love hiding in cardboard and dark corners.
- Vacuum webs and egg sacs immediately.
- Keep porch lights off—light attracts insects, which attract spiders.

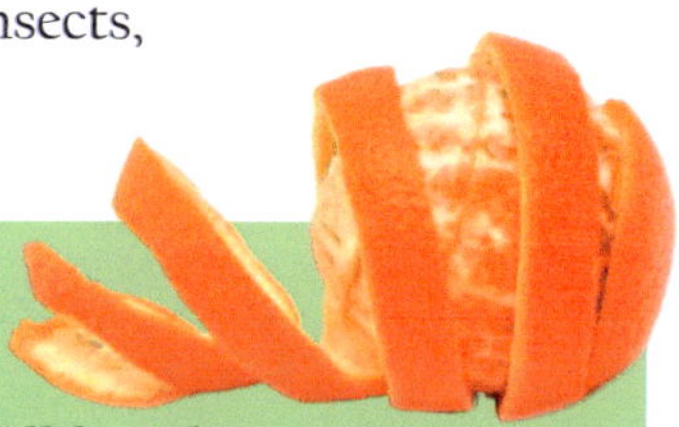

Bonus Tips:

- Use a chestnut or conker in corners (folklore, but many swear by it).
- Close blinds or curtains at night to keep bugs away from light.
- Dust ceiling corners regularly—no web, no squatters.

When to Call a Pro:
If you're seeing large spiders regularly or suspect a venomous species, call a pest expert to inspect and treat safely.

CHAPTER 8
WASPS — THE AGGRESSIVE INVADERS

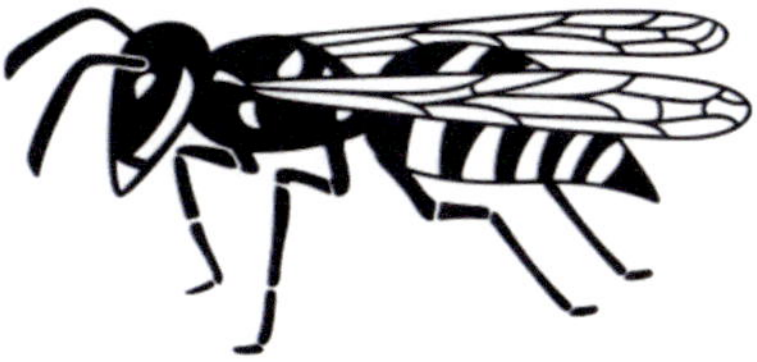

Unlike bees, wasps don't mess around. These territorial stingers can turn outdoor spaces into no-go zones. Let's reclaim your porch and patio.

Why They Come:
Wasps are drawn to protein early in the season and sugar later. Trash, food, and eaves make perfect nesting zones.

Natural Remedies:

- **Peppermint Oil:** Wasps can't stand it. Mix with water and dish soap as a spray.
- **Fake Nest:** Wasps are territorial and avoid areas with another nest. Hang a decoy.
- **Clove, Geranium & Lemongrass Oil Mix:** A powerful anti-wasp spray combo.
- **Vinegar Trap:** Mix vinegar, sugar, and dish soap in a bottle to trap them.

Lifestyle & Prevention Tips:

- Cover trash tightly and clean bins.
- Avoid leaving sugary drinks or meats outside.
- Inspect and seal cracks and holes in siding rooflines.

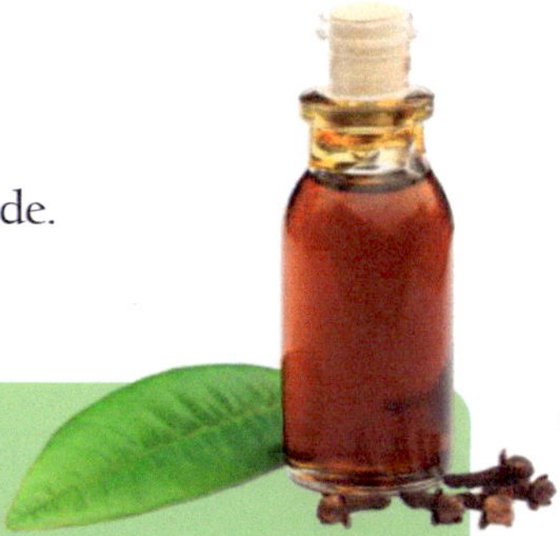

Bonus Tips:

- Hang paper bags shaped like nests under eaves.
- Place cucumber peels near entry points.
- Knock down small nests early in the season (wear protection).

When to Call a Pro:
Large nests or aggressive behavior = time for trained professionals. Wasps can be dangerous if disturbed.

CHAPTER 9
BED BUGS — THE SNEAKY BLOODSUCKERS

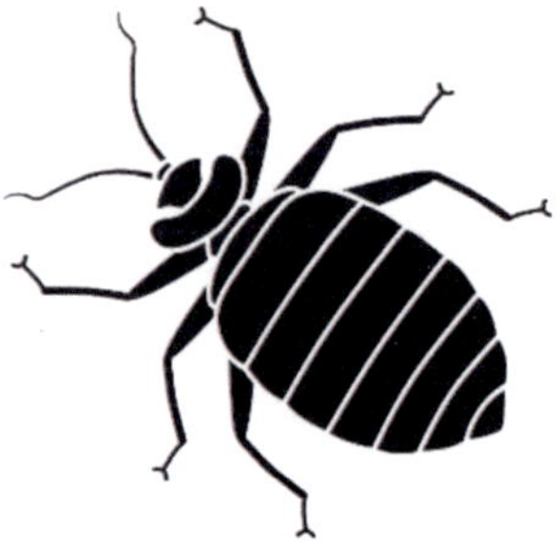

Ah yes, the stuff of itchy nightmares. Bed bugs are stealthy, persistent, and incredibly frustrating. But you can fight back—naturally and smartly.

Why They Come:
They hitchhike on luggage, clothing, or furniture. Once in, they hide in mattresses, bed frames, and cracks.

Natural Remedies:

- **Steam Cleaning:** High heat kills all stages. Use on mattresses and furniture.
- **Diatomaceous Earth:** Dust along baseboards and bed frames.
- **Tea Tree Oil Spray:** Mix with water and spray on affected areas.
- **Lavender Oil:** A natural repellent and sleep aid—win-win.

Lifestyle & Prevention Tips:

- Don't bring home used furniture without inspection.
- Use mattress and box spring encasements.
- Reduce clutter near the bed.

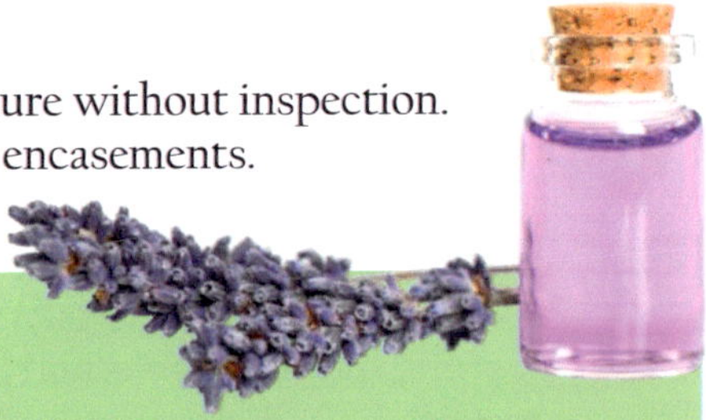

Bonus Tips:

- Place interceptors under bed legs to trap bugs.
- Wash bedding on hot and dry on high heat.
- Vacuum seams and crevices every few days during treatment.

When to Call a Pro:
Bed bugs are notoriously hard to eliminate alone. If sightings persist, bring in a licensed pest control expert with heat or chemical treatments.

CHAPTER 10

TICKS — THE TINY OUTDOOR HITCHHIKERS

Ticks don't bite—they latch. And they can carry serious diseases like Lyme. Protecting your home and pets from these parasites is a must.

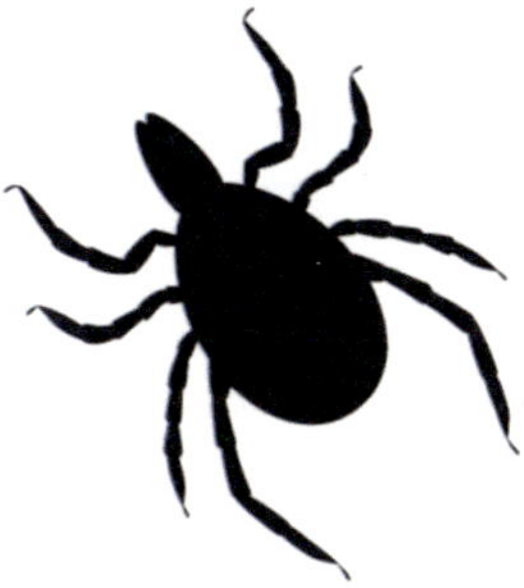

Why They Come:
They wait in tall grass, leaf piles, and wooded areas, looking to hitch a ride.

Natural Remedies:

- **Eucalyptus & Lemon Oil Spray:** Safe on clothing and shoes.
- **Cedar Oil Spray:** Effective and pet-safe.
- **Diatomaceous Earth:** Spread around lawn edges and pet paths.
- **Apple Cider Vinegar in Pet Water:** A few drops (with vet approval) may deter ticks.

Lifestyle & Prevention Tips:

- Keep lawns trimmed and clear debris.
- Create a barrier of gravel or wood chips between yard and woods.
- Inspect pets and people after time outdoors.

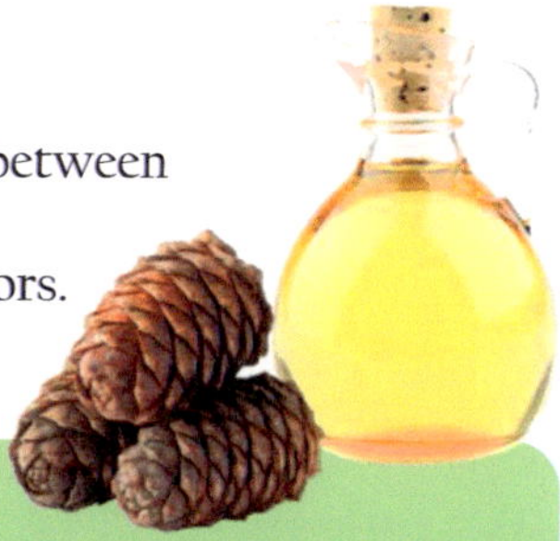

Bonus Tips:

- Tumble clothes on high heat for 10 mins after outdoor exposure.
- Avoid sitting directly on grass in wooded areas.
- Use tick repellent collars for pets.

When to Call a Pro:
Persistent tick sightings or if your yard backs up to woods or fields, a pro can apply safe perimeter treatments.

CHAPTER 11
SILVERFISH — THE PAPER-EATING SHADOWS

Silverfish are nocturnal, quick, and love humid places. They won't bite—but they'll munch on paper, books, and cereal. Let's evict them.

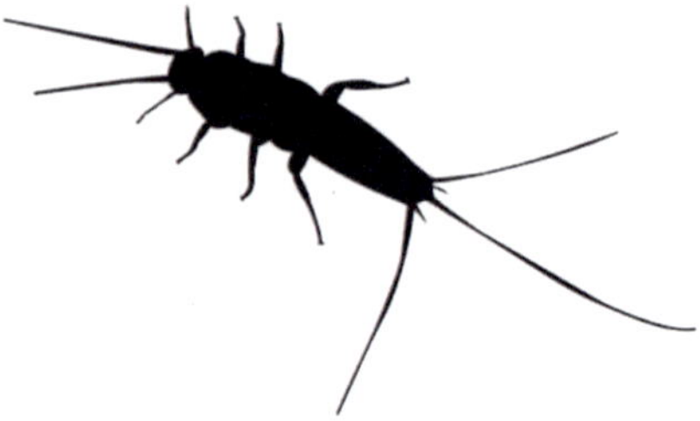

Why They Come:
They thrive in humidity and love starches like glue, paper, and grains.

Natural Remedies:

- **Diatomaceous Earth:** Sprinkle under sinks, near baseboards, and behind appliances.
- **Cucumber Peels:** Repel silverfish naturally.
- **Lavender Sachets:** Fresh-smelling deterrents for closets and drawers.
- **Cloves:** Strong scent keeps them away from food and papers.

Lifestyle & Prevention Tips:

- Use a dehumidifier in bathrooms and basements.
- Store papers in plastic bins.
- Fix leaky pipes.

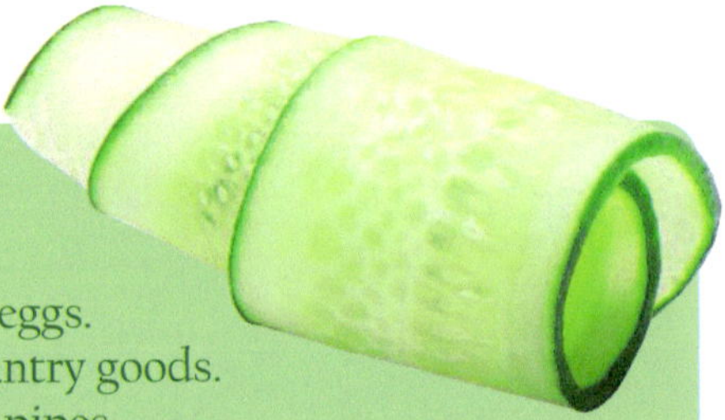

Bonus Tips:

- Vacuum regularly to pick up eggs.
- Use airtight containers for pantry goods.
- Seal cracks around walls and pipes.

When to Call a Pro:
If silverfish are destroying valuable items or appear in large numbers, pest pros can target hidden areas effectively.

CHAPTER 12
MOTHS — THE SILENT FABRIC RAIDERS

If your favorite sweater has mystery holes, moths may be the culprit. These quiet invaders prefer dark closets and wool—but you can keep them at bay naturally.

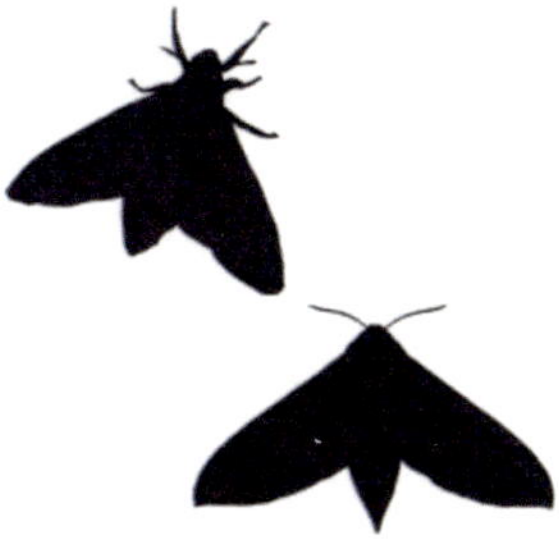

Why They Come:
They're drawn to natural fibers, food crumbs, and undisturbed closets.

Natural Remedies:

- **Cedar Blocks or Hangers:** A classic moth repellent.
- **Lavender Sachets:** Smell good and send moths away.
- **Vinegar Wipe-Downs:** Clean shelves and drawers with diluted vinegar.
- **Freezer Method:** Freeze affected clothes for 72 hours to kill larvae.

Lifestyle & Prevention Tips:

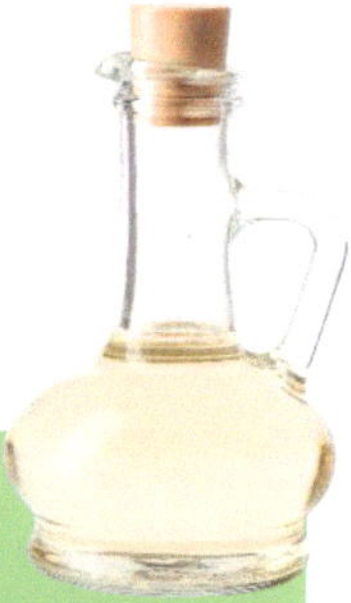

- Wash clothes before storing.
- Store seasonal items in airtight bags or bins.
- Keep closets clean and vacuumed.

Bonus Tips:

- Rotate clothes regularly—moths like undisturbed garments.
- Use essential oil sprays (lavender, rosemary, eucalyptus).
- Inspect vintage or thrift finds before bringing them in.

When to Call a Pro:
If moths spread beyond clothing to pantry or textiles, pros can eliminate hidden eggs and stop the cycle.

EXTRA BONUS SECTION
HEALTHY HOME HABITS FOR A PEST-FREE LIFE

Pest control starts with lifestyle. These habits work across the board for preventing almost every common bug:

- **Declutter regularly.** Pests love hiding in untouched spaces.
- **Fix leaks fast.** Dampness attracts all kinds of creepy crawlies.
- **Seal entry points.** Caulk cracks, patch screens, and weatherproof doors.
- **Store food properly.** Use sealed glass or plastic containers.
- **Clean drains.** Sink gunk feeds drain flies and other pests.
- **Vacuum weekly.** Especially under beds, appliances, and rugs.
- **Use essential oils.** Peppermint, lavender, citronella, and eucalyptus are multi-purpose repellents.
- **Inspect bags and shoes.** Especially after travel or outdoor time.
- **Practice yard hygiene.** No standing water, no untrimmed grass, and no firewood piles next to the home.

RESOURCES & FURTHER READING

Looking to dive deeper into natural pest control, safe household ingredients, or eco-friendly living? Below are some trusted sources and organizations that support the remedies and prevention tips in this book:

Trusted Information Sources

- **National Pesticide Information Center (NPIC)** – www.npic.orst.edu
  Reliable, science-based information about pesticides, safety, and alternatives.
- **Environmental Protection Agency (EPA) – Safer Choice** – www.epa.gov/saferchoice
  Products and ingredients deemed safer for humans and the environment.
- **Beyond Pesticides** – www.beyondpesticides.org
  Non-profit promoting organic and least-toxic pest solutions.

Natural Remedy Support

- **Rodale Institute** – www.rodaleinstitute.org
  Leaders in organic and sustainable living—great for natural gardening tips.
- **The Old Farmer's Almanac** – www.almanac.com/pest-control
  Homegrown solutions for seasonal pests and prevention techniques.

DIY & Ingredient Guides

- **Healthline Natural Cleaning Guide** – www.healthline.com
  Great breakdowns of natural cleaning ingredients like vinegar, baking soda, and lemon.
- **National Center for Biotechnology Information (NCBI)** – www.ncbi.nlm.nih.gov
  Scientific studies on essential oils, boric acid, and plant-based pest deterrents.

ABOUT THE AUTHOR

Misti Coyle is a licensed pest control professional with over 17 years of field experience and multiple industry certifications. She's passionate about helping families take back their homes—naturally. Misti believes pest control doesn't have to mean chemicals everywhere, and her heart is in empowering others through education, clean habits, and the occasional peppermint oil spray.

Made in the USA
Monee, IL
05 November 2026

67377491R00017